# *Nursing School Survival Guide:*
# Stress and Time Management

By Shari Lynn Kvidahl, RN

# Table of Contents

| | |
|---|---|
| Stress and Anxiety in Nursing School | 1 |
|     The Anxiety Budget | 1 |
|     Rules of the Anxiety Budget | 2 |
|     The Deposit | 2 |
|     Making a Withdraw | 3 |
|     Replenishing | 4 |
|     Managing the Stress of Grades in Nursing School | 7 |
|         Building a Grade Predictor | 9 |
| Time Management in Nursing School | 14 |
|     What does Florence Nightingale Think? | 15 |
|     Time Management Techniques | 16 |
|     Time Wasters | 18 |
| References | 21 |
| About the Author | 23 |

# Stress and Anxiety in Nursing School

It goes without saying, nursing school is stressful. A recent study published in *The Journal of Nursing Education and Practice* indicated stress in nursing school is not limited to the country of origin (Jones, Hansen, Kaddoura, Schwab-McCoy, & Tocchini, 2018). Additionally, stress is more prevalent in healthcare students than in students seeking non-healthcare related fields. However, the critical factor in this study was the new understanding of the importance of stress managing activities. As individuals who participated in yoga, exercise, camping or being outdoors had significantly lower stress levels than those, who did not. I tell you all of this to inform you of your personal anxiety budget and how to manage your budget to buy yourself the least stressful nursing education.

## The Anxiety Budget

Stress exists on a continuum. It is not a linear practice, really. You become stressed; your stress levels rise. You become relaxed; your stress levels lower. With that said, the power to become stressed is yours and yours alone. Not to suggest anxiety as a diagnosis isn't real, because it is, and it is treatable. In no way is the information shared about an anxiety budget a substitute for medicine or counseling about personal anxiety. Instead, the anxiety budget is designed to augment traditional counseling and even medication for cases of anxiety seen in nursing, nursing school and healthcare in general.

## Rules of the Anxiety Budget
1. Each day you awaken with the same deposit into your anxiety budget.
2. As time progresses in nursing school, your deposit grows.
3. Each task or unpredicted event has an associated 'cost' from your budget.
4. Ultimately, you determine the price of each associated event.
5. When you fully empty your anxiety bank, you go into panic mode or have an anxiety attack.
6. Much like your bank account, only you can authorize the spending of anxiety 'points.'
7. It is possible to add to your anxiety budget through acts of personal self-care and relaxation exercises.

## The Deposit.

Many people in healthcare can debate when the day begins. For those who work first shift, the day starts at midnight. Nurses who work the night shift, they might consider the day to start at five o'clock when they awaken for their shifts. No matter what shift you work, or when you mainly sleep. When you awaken, for the purpose of the anxiety budget, is the beginning of a new day. Each day is a clean slate. Matter of fact that is so important you should say it out loud. *A new day is a clean slate.*

You cannot continue to harbor the shortcomings of yesterday in nursing school (or life). It is difficult enough to continue to learn and grow, but to hold out for yesterday's problems will not progress you any further today. Take what you can learn from them, leave all the rest behind, you are too busy to carry that around with you.

## Making a Withdraw

Every part of your day requires a withdraw from the anxiety bank. As time progresses some tasks require far less of a withdraw than before. For instance, a one-year-old children withdraw from the anxiety bank for walking from the bedroom to the bathroom would be significantly higher than a college student. The discrepancy is because a college student has done it for years upon years and has built up confidence and comfort in performing the task. To put this into the context of your journey in nursing school, the anxiety you feel when practicing the insertion of an indwelling urinary catheter for the first time will be significantly less than that experienced on the one-hundredth time. Due to the familiarity gained by performing the task several times.

When making a withdraw, I suggest you ask yourself *"do I have the budget for this?"* Don't spend your time or budget on frivolous things like what Susy-Jo-Que thinks about the girl who sits behind her and asks too many questions. You do not have the budget for that, save those 'points' and use them for something more important (like a pop-quiz). It is effortless to waste your anxiety budget on silly things like gossip, worrying over a single point lost on a test or the troubles of yesterday. As I stated before, you must let them go to save your stress for the more important things.

## Replenishing

The next question I often get is, *how do I get my anxiety 'points' back?* There are a significant number of ways to replenish anxiety budget points. They require personal attention and relaxation. Personal time is something nursing students are taught to ignore. The same study in *The Journal of Nursing Education and Practice* found students who used relaxation techniques and gave themselves personal care had lower levels of stress and anxiety than those who did not (Jones, Hansen, Kaddoura, Schwab-McCoy, & Tocchini, 2018). I have included a list of some relaxation techniques to help you, and some self-care practices to rejuvenate your anxiety budget.

Paint your toenails, many nursing schools do not allow students to paint fingernails for health and safety reasons, but toenails are fair game. Invite some friends over and study while painting nails.

Have a glass of wine, once a week. It is an excellent way to unwind and according to the American Heart

Association, promotes heart health (American Heart Association, 2014). You are becoming a nurse, with a heart of gold. Better keep it healthy.

- Go for a walk, even if it is just around campus. Commit to going for a walk once a day, or a few times a week. You can do this in-between classes or go with friends and make a group of it.

- Make a weekly meeting for coffee or ice-cream. Not to suggest packing on the "freshman 15" but making a set, organized time to meet with your friends and catch up on the (non-nursing school related) ways of the world can improve the status of your mental health. Remember there is life before nursing school, there is life in nursing school, and there is life after nursing school.

- Take a bubble bath. Warm bubble baths are a great way to relax muscles and rejuvenate the body (Runtastic Team, 2015). *Runtastic*, a website dedicated to running enthusiasts suggest a concoction of 1 spoon of each shampoo, coconut oil, and Epsom salt mixed with a bathtub of water and 5-8 drops of lavender oil.

- Watch your favorite movie or show. CAUTION: Television can be a time sucker. Set limits and stick with those limits. See more in the time management section of this book.

- Take a nap. I can't stress enough how much sleep contributes to stress hormone production. A study in 2015 found a decreased amount of norepinephrine in those who had taken a nap, even when experiencing poor sleep, the previous night (Faraut, et al., 2015). Remember there is a direct correlation between norepinephrine, stress, and depression; making a small 30-45 min nap a great de-stressing tool.

- Infuse essential oils. Lavender and Rosemary have been shown to decrease cortisol levels when inhaled (Atsumi & Tonosaki, 2007). An infuser in your bedroom is a beautiful edition or add a small number of drops of essential oil to cotton balls and leave them out while studying.

- Listen to music. Pick any music you like and jam out. Sing along, like no one is watching. Trust me, anyone who hears you will think you are crazy because you decided to add going to college to your already busy schedule, not because you are singing to the music.

- Deep breathing exercises. There are many apps on your phone which can help you to keep rhythm with your breathing. Blowing bubbles also help to keep breathing even and low.

While this list is not inclusive of what you can do to replenish your anxiety bank, they are starters and ideas. Everyone has things they find more relaxing. Some may enjoy fishing, camping, and biking; while others may see it just as relaxing to stay inside and bake some cookies. Whatever it is that makes you whole, do that.

## Managing the Stress of Grades in Nursing School

The stress of grades can be crucial to many students in nursing school. It is common, and an ancient practice to pit students against each other based on grades. For example, in some nursing schools' students with the highest grade point average (GPA) are rewarded with choice clinical rotations. However, this reinforces the notion that only some nurses survive or that only the best nurses are good nurses; this is not true. Many nursing schools are embracing the idea of different nurses.

Many aspects of nursing are different, rather than wrong. For instance, when asking a long-term care nurse about the expiration of a single-use liter of normal saline for a patient vs. an acute care nurse from a hospital. The long-term care nurse will tell you the bottle is good for twenty-four hours if kept in the patient's room and describe the facility protocol to labeling. However, the acute-care nurse will tell you it is only good for the time used, and once the task is performed, it should be discarded. Which is wrong? Neither. They are both right for their setting and the particulars of their practice. Embrace differences, ask why, rather than accept one as wrong. It is understanding the why, which leads to the real knowledge needed in nursing.

How does all this play into managing the stress of grades in nursing school? Because the most critical thing a nursing student can do is to remediate the questions missed on tests, quizzes and in lecture. These practices lead to an understanding of why. Many times, under the exemplary stress of nursing school we begin to believe we can fight the answers to be right. Resist this urge. Remediate to understand why the other response was the most right. After all, the National Council Licensure Examination (NCLEX) is a test with all the right answers provided. With only one solution being the 'rightest'.

Another way to prevent unnecessary anxiety about grades is to establish a grade predictor. Creating the spreadsheet can be a daunting task, but I have included instructions. I suggest and endorse establishing your predictor at the beginning of your class. Doing so allows you to have a good understanding of your placement in class as it progresses. Once you have established a single sheet, you can copy and paste throughout the semester or time you are in nursing school. I like to build mine on google documents, because of the web-based accessibility it gives.

## Building a Grade Predictor

Start by creating, or logging into, your google account. Then open google docs. Click on the "new document" icon.

*Figure 1: Google New Document Button*

Then, select the "Untitled spreadsheet" located at the top left-hand side of the screen. Change that to "Grade Predictor." You can change the name to whatever you would like, but make sure you can remember it at a later date.

 Untitled spreadsheet

File   Edit   View   Insert

Then in box A1, you need to place the word "assignment." A2 should be labeled "grade" and finally A3 "worth." When completed it should

| | A | B | C |
|---|---|---|---|
| 1 | Assignment | Grade | Worth |

look like the area below. Center the text, if it suits you.

*Figure 2: Names on the specific rows of the grade predictor.*

The rest of this tutorial is dependent on your program and class. However, I am going to fill out our demonstration sheet following my own class assignments for my bachelors; this is where you would look at the syllabus for your class. (No, the syllabus is not just for making coasters during study sessions, it is a treasured piece of information)

The curriculum should outline the plan for the class. If your program has an online grading system, you may be able to copy and paste from the grading system. Please fill in the assignment column with the assignments for this class.

We will be skipping filling out the 'grade' column right now, as you shouldn't have any grades to enter here. We will fill out the 'worth' column. The 'C"' column is for the grade the assignment is worth. In the final cell (the one after the last 'worth' grade in column 'C') place the following function, replacing # with the number of the last grade; in the case of this demonstration it is cell 25, so I would put in C25

# =SUM (C2:C#)

The sum feature will total the column and give the total points available for the entire class; and is helpful information, but alone it gets you nothing. You can start by predicting your grades based on your GPA, which is useful. If you have a 4.0 GPA, give yourself a perfect score all the way down the column. However, for the rest of us reading this book we may need to do some math! If your GPA is a 3.67 is a 90-93% on an undergraduate scale. Multiply the possible grade by your current GPA to find the predicted score. Using the lower end allows for more natural representation of your growth. Using the upper end, well that leads to excess anxiety. I will use 90% for my example. Sum the "grade" column when you have finished. The result should look something like this:

| | A | B | C |
|---|---|---|---|
| 1 | Assignment | Grade | Worth |
| 2 | Discussion 1.1 | 18 | 20 |
| 3 | Discussion 1.2 | 18 | 20 |
| 4 | Assignment 1 | 90 | 100 |
| 5 | Discussion 2.1 | 18 | 20 |
| 6 | Discussion 2.2 | 18 | 20 |
| 7 | Assignment 2 | 90 | 100 |
| 8 | Discussion 3.1 | 18 | 20 |
| 9 | Discussion 3.2 | 18 | 20 |
| 10 | Assignment 3 | 90 | 100 |
| 11 | Discussion 4.1 | 18 | 20 |
| 12 | Discussion 4.2 | 18 | 20 |
| 13 | Assigment 4 | 90 | 100 |
| 14 | Discussion 5.1 | 18 | 20 |
| 15 | Discussion 5.2 | 18 | 20 |
| 16 | Assignment 5 | 90 | 100 |
| 17 | Discussion 6.1 | 18 | 20 |
| 18 | Discussion 6.2 | 18 | 20 |
| 19 | Assignment 6 | 90 | 100 |
| 20 | Discussion 7.1 | 18 | 20 |
| 21 | Discussion 7.2 | 18 | 20 |
| 22 | Assignment 7 | 90 | 100 |
| 23 | Discussion 8.1 | 18 | 20 |
| 24 | Discussion 8.2 | 18 | 20 |
| 25 | Assignment 8 | 90 | 100 |
| 26 | **TOTAL** | **1008** | **1120** |

*Figure 3: Grade Predictor before adding percentile function*

The last part is to add the percentile function; this is a relatively easy task. Select the cell to the right of the total of the 'worth' column and enter "=(B#/C#)*100" where the # is the number of your total column. The examples are row 26.

As the semester goes and assignments are completed, place the grades in the grade column, overwrite the existing (predicted) grade. When complete, you will have a clearer picture. It is specially helpful if your professor takes a little while to put the grades in the system.

# Time Management in Nursing School

Time management is a crucial skill for daily life, let alone for nursing school. Developing a strong time management technique, one that is effective for you personally, will last you well into your practice and beyond. I find it is not enough to have time in the day, but rather it is the understanding of what to do with the time available. Excellent time management is like a road trip.

When deciding to take a trip, it is essential to know where you are going. The same is true of managing the hours in a day. Identifying the objectives or goals for the day is essential. Set small goals, and broad targets. Today's goal may be to change the laundry over to the dryer, or it could be to write a five-page paper. It all depends on where you are going. The next thing you need to decide is how you are getting there.

If we are going on a road trip, are we taking your car or mine? Will we take a plane, train or bus? If you are planning out your day, will you use a calendar, a planner, or an electronic agenda? The choice is yours. Choose a planning style that works best for you and your situation. If you are single and living alone; you may not need an electronic journal. If you remember best by writing, consider a planner. Experiment with one or all and remember one may not be the only solution. I use an electronic planner through a web-based service and a physical planner. The web-based planner allows for family members to link into the planner and view events.

### What does Florence Nightingale think?

Throughout nursing school, it is vital to reflect on the thoughts of Florence Nightingale. About time management, the *Lady with a Lamp* is very opinionated. Namely women, when reflecting on the time, nurses were primarily women. Because of this, Nightingale often uses women and nurses interchangeably; or at least this is relevant to interpretation today. Nightingale wrote in her book *Cassandra and Suggestions for Thought*, a bit of understanding on why time management is so important.

*"Why do people sit up so late, or, more rarely, get up so early? Not because the day is not long enough, but because they have no time in the day to themselves."*
(Nightingale, 1991)

Nightingale references the rationale for getting up early or going to bed late have more to do with having no time left in the day for personal time. Rather than needing more time in the day. As a nursing student, you will never be at a loss for completing tasks. The day will end with plenty more to do tomorrow and the next day. That is why nursing school is not a three-week course.

## Time Management Techniques

Knowing how to tie your shoe keeps it on your foot. Time management is no different. If you want to maintain control of your time, it is good to know how to manage it. Below is a list of helpful techniques to make the most of your day. These will help you to squeeze the most out of the 16 hours (or 20) you are awake.

- **Set Goals.** The goal can be broad like 'study for A&P test' but be sure to break it down into digestible chunks. For instance, you may break this down into each chapter, or unit, covered and then into the individual subject you feel may be included. Once the goals are achieved, mark it off the list. Keep a LOSTT list. LOSTT stands for List Of Stuff To-do Today. The list of things that can't possibly wait for tomorrow. Don't add stuff to this list unless it expires, or someone dies at midnight. This list is designed to be the hard-stop, if you will, for the day.
- **Say no to Extra Tasks.** I keep a robust 12-16-hour notice policy. Please, do not ask me to do anything without at least a 12-hour notice. You should be able to project the tasks you need to perform at least 12-hours in advance. Much of nursing, as you will find out, is fortune telling in a way (or predicting, if that tickles your fancy more).
- **Delegate.** Ask yourself 'Self, does the person who performs this task NEED to be me?" If the answer is no, then you should delegate it to someone

else who isn't in nursing school to do. Practicing now is a good for when you are a nurse and need to figure out what to delegate — things like baking cookies for your son's bake sale. Trust me; the grocery store can do that task. Some things, like sewing up your daughter's teddy bear, well those are more important than you do. Weight your personal beliefs and act accordingly.

- **Give Tasks a Time Limit.** Getting up in the morning, set a time limit on how long you will take to be ready. Tell yourself; you need to be prepared in a fixed period of time, and stick with it. I can tell you, I left home without socks before, because my time to spend on that task was up. The same is true for you, set a time limit on tasks. Clearer expectation on time expendature will also allow you to better schedule tasks into your routine.
- **Do a Time Evaluation.** Audit yourself, see where your time goes. Some apps will let you see how much of your time is being spent on various programs. Spend a week and count up where your time went. An alternate version of this requires a paper plate and some candy or berries. Divide the paper plate into eight sections, kind of like you slice a pizza. Label each section after a role or task you must perform; remember to add nursing school to the pie. Some other fields might be work, family, caregiver, personal time, transportation, study, etc. Then add those berries or candy to each section. One berry, or

candy, to represent an hour of your day. You will soon see where most of your time goes.

While these are not an inclusive list, it is important to remember that your time must work for you. You are not a passenger in nursing school, but an active participant. For instance, when you are waiting between classes. There is a perfect opportunity to complete some flash cards. Many online sources have flashcards, or you can make your own. Instead of surfing Facebook while you wait for the transit, consider reading your textbook instead? Making the most of your time is one way you save up additional 15-minute increments of the day to milk an extra hour out.

## Time Wasters

It seems foolish to fail to mention the things a student can do to waste time. Here are some nonproductive uses for your time. This list is of unproductive tasks you can perform in nursing school, but it is a good deal of them. These are also good ideas as you move forward with your nursing career.

- **Social Media.** The Nielsen Group (2018), a leader in research on social media and television has found at the end of quarter one in 2018 nearly half of the day is spent interacting with media in the United States. Of this time, four hours was spent watching television and another three on social media apps like Snapchat or Facebook. Cutting these activities out of your day, well that will give you twice as much time in a day.

- **Drama.** Save the drama for your llama. If you have a llama, give it to its momma. Gossip and cliques are great for *Game of Thrones*, but there is no need for a red wedding in your nursing school, or in the nursing profession either. Set proper boundaries for yourself in terms of interactions with other nursing students and friends. Be mindful of the adverse effects, not only on your time, on your psyche when engaging in drama or gossip as a matter of fact. Dr. Nicholas Emler found, in a study of 300 individuals, 80% of their time was spent discussion other people; and more specifically the habits of other people (Macrae, 2009). Save the time, don't gossip.
- **Web-browsing.** Apps like Pinterest and Yahoo make it easy to avoid the tasks we need to be completing because it is all too enticing to see one more article or one more pin. Web-browsing is a dangerous game for a nursing student to fall prey. Try using a screen-limiting application. Also, be wary of Netflix. It is easy to lose hours of your day to meaningless content, at least when you compare the content to the studying you need to be doing.

- **Parties.** I am not suggesting you decline your mother-in-law's invitation to Christmas dinner. However, it is a waste of time to participate in activities like 'keggers' or drinking games. Avoid the bar; instead have study groups. The people attending will understand your struggles, and you will form friendships that will be much more lasting when you become a nurse and can't be hungover and calculating drip rates.
- **Cell Phones.** Cell phones, almost everyone has one. Most of them are smart. Limit your screen times for the same reasons previously mentioned under web-browsing. It is helpful to be able to look things up, and applications like NCLEX-Mastery are great study resources. While I endorse the idea of using apps like Quizzlet during your downtime, stay away from time burners like Facebook, Snapchat or Whatsapp. These do not provide you any educational benefit and just steal the time you need to get things done that matter to you.

# References

American Heart Association. (2014, August 14). *Alcohol and heart health*. Retrieved from American Heart Association: https://www.heart.org/en/healthy-living/healthy-eating/eat-smart/nutrition-basics/alcohol-and-heart-health#

Atsumi, T., & Tonosaki, K. (2007, February 28). Smelling lavendar and rosemary increase free radical scavenging activity and decreases cortisol level in saliva. *Psychiatry Research*, 89-96. doi:10.1016/j.psychres.2005.12.012

Faraut, B., Nakib, S., Drogou, C., Elbaz, M., Sauvet, F., De Bandt, J.-P., & Leger, D. (2015, March 1). Napping reverses the salivary interleukin-6 and urinary norepinephrine changes induced by sleep restriction. *Journal of Clinical Endocrinology & Metabolism, 100*(3), 416-426. doi:10.1210/jc.2014-2566

Jones, R., Hansen, M., Kaddoura, M., Schwab-McCoy, A., & Tocchini, K. (2018, May 29). The incidence of nursing students' perceived stress and burnout levels at a private university in California. *Journal of Nursing Education and Practice, 8*(10), 138-151. doi:10.5430/jnep.v8n10p138

Macrae, F. (2009, September 8). You'll never guess what... We spend 80% of our time gossiping. *The Daily Mail*. Retrieved from https://www.dailymail.co.uk/sciencetech/article-1211863/Youll-guess--We-spend-80-cent-time-gossiping.html

Nightingale, F. (1991). *Cassandra and Suggestions for Thought.* New York: Routledge.

Runtastic Team. (2015, August 1). *The power of a bubble bath: Reduce stress & relax your muscles*. Retrieved from Runtastic: https://www.runtastic.com/blog/en/reduce-stress-and-relax-your-muscles/

The Nielsen Group. (2018, July 31). *Time flies: US adults now spend nearly half a day interacting with media*. Retrieved from The Nielsen Group: https://www.nielsen.com/us/en/insights/news/2018/time-flies-us-adults-now-spend-nearly-half-a-day-interacting-with-media.print.html

# About the Author

Shari Lynn Kvidahl is a Registered Nurse and Adjunct Instructor in Cedar Rapids, Iowa. Nursing was the third career for Shari. First she joined the Army out of high school, later to attend Kirkwood Community College in pursuit of an associate degree in Equine Science. Then she would attend Kaplan University to gain her associate degree in Nursing. With a background in long-term care, she currently practices at St. Luke's – Unity Point Hospital in Cedar Rapids. She enjoys being the 'different' instructor at Kirkwood Community College's nursing program and is often found in the Foundations to Nursing and Introduction to Nursing Lab sections; she will be the one with a bow. A mother of three, diligent wife and continual student. Her advice on time management and stress comes from the juggle of two jobs, three children and aspiring to gain a graduate degree.

www.ingramcontent.com/pod-product-compliance
Lightning Source LLC
Chambersburg PA
CBHW031941170526
45157CB00008B/3265